DIABETES
MADE
BETTER

Live, Feel, and Look Good
While Managing Your Diabetes

Danielle Batiste

DIABETES MADE BETTER

Live, Feel, and Look Good
While Managing Your Diabetes

DANIELLE BATISTE

ISBN: 978-0-578-32650-4
Library of Congress Control Number

D & B Publishing Co.
Newport News, VA
www.daniellebatiste.com

FOREWORD

My initial encounter with Danielle Batiste was on a video screen. COVID19 had closed our primary care practice to all in-person visits and, daily, I struggled to find that human connection with patients without the help of a handshake or other physical contact. With Danielle Batiste, it was easy. Her passion, energy, and humanity seemed to jump out of the screen. I was eager to read her books, the first of which I devoured in one captivated sitting.

In **Diabetes Made Better**, Danielle Batiste does it again. Her can- do mindset and pragmatic approach to living with Type 2 diabetes is a refreshing change from the usual medical jargon found in "patient education" literature. Batiste moves adeptly from science to compassion to personal testimony that is engaging and "real." Through a vulnerable narrative, she opens a world of understanding through personal experiences beginning the day of her own medical diagnosis.

From a good night's sleep to a pedicure, travel planning to yeast infections, Batiste shares her personal victories and struggles with a humility and zeal that will inspire diabetics, family members, and health care providers alike. What surprised me about this book is how Ms. Batiste uses her own story to educate and empower people. "Everyone is different," she writes and in so doing, she gives the reader permission to create his/her own narrative for health and wellbeing.

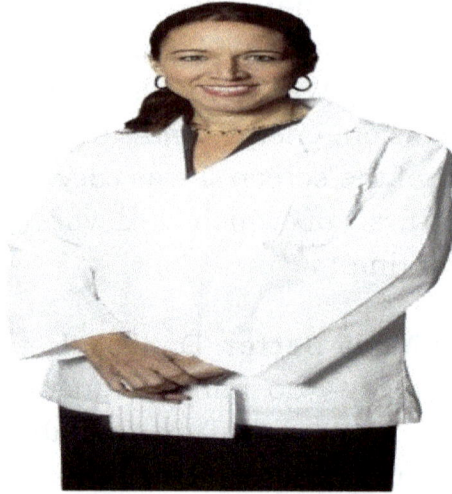

Photo Credit: Hampton Roads Physician, Good Deeds Winter 2015

Susan B. Girois, MD MPH
FACP Women's Health
Medical Director Primary
Care Physician
Hampton VA Medical Center

Danielle's personal knowledge and insight as an advocate for healthy living despite being a diabetic are impressive. Recently I met with my doctor to discuss my numbers and what deems a person a diabetic. I used Danielle's knowledge to see if my doctor was being transparent with me. Her knowledge prepared me for what questions to ask.

Danielle helped me understand and navigate diabetes. Because of her, I was able to be an active participant in my treatment plan, so much so that my lifestyle change kept me from being prescribed any medication.

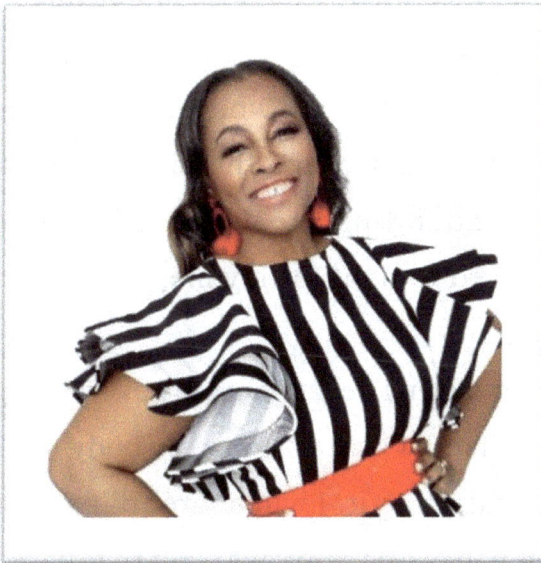

Photo Credit: Cheryl Pullins

Cheryl Pullins, CEO Her Iconic Empire
Award-Winning International Speaker Founder, Iconic Persona Agency | Transforming Ordinary into Iconic

PRELUDE

I will never forget my reaction when I was diagnosed as a Type 2 diabetic. I went into denial, which was the easiest thing to do, and seemed to be the safest place to go. I ate what I wanted, did what I wanted, and lived life like I did before I was diagnosed. What seemed to be the easiest thing to do and the safest place to go meant that my glucose levels were out of control. I did not have a clue on how to handle the dysfunction, so I continued to do nothing.

After going through this for a while, I realized I could not live like that forever. I was letting the disease win and quitting, and defeat are not my nature. I fought for my country, but I somehow refused to fight for my life.

Enough was enough. I began learning everything on my own. The first thing I did was learn how my body worked and how diabetes was affecting it. I will share that shocking truth in the following pages and empower you to take control of your life.

Diabetes is not a death sentence unless you allow it to be.

I started paying more attention to what I ate, read labels, and received the correct numbers from my doctor. What I hated the most was pricking my finger and the way I had to live. Another major challenge for me was getting out there and exercising. (No, exercise is not something that everyone enjoys.)

I lost 40 pounds and that is when the fighter in me began. I knew then that I wanted to help others feel and accomplish the same thing I did.

As diabetics, we tend to go through a roller coaster of thoughts and emotions. Some days it's Lord, why me? Other times we want to give up but we're ready to take on the world and fight. We are insanely happy when our A1C is great, but insanely upset three months later when the number is higher. This is the nature of the life of a diabetic.

If I can be a source of encouragement, I want to challenge you to stop beating yourself up. Reprogram your mind to one of an athlete. One of my mantras is:

> *I am doing what I must do to live. I will not have any number determine if diabetes will regulate my life. I am in control and making life changes to enhance my life and health.*

As the CEO of Diabetes Made Better, LLC, I am on a mission to empower and educate diabetics to live, feel, and look good without living for the numbers. In this book, it is not my intention to be politically correct but to be politically me. To take better care of ourselves, you need to know the following fact from the Centers for Disease Control[1] (this is not a scare tactic):

Diabetes is the 7th leading cause of death versus heart disease which is the #1 cause.

I would be absent-minded if I did not also warn you to be careful and mindful of how you protect yourself in COVID-19. Diabetes and other diseases make us more vulnerable to catching viruses and slower to recover and heal from them. Please take extra precautions for your safety such as wearing your masks, frequently washing your hands, and disinfecting as well as minimizing your exposure to high-risk activities. The Covid-19 vaccine is an invaluable tool to protect the health and safety of Americans and end the pandemic that has taken a staggering toll on people living with diabetes.

Diabetes is not a death sentence unless you allow it to be.

---

[1] "Leading Causes of Death." *Cdc.Gov*, 1 Mar. 2021, https://www.cdc.gov/nchs/fastats/leading-causes-of-death.htm.

Table of Contents

WHAT IS DIABETES?

Danielle Batiste

I n this chapter, I am going to talk about what diabetes is and the different types. A lot of people have a diagnosis but do not research what type of diabetes they have and what they need to do to maintain and control it properly. The following information is given to help you make informed decisions when it comes to your health.

What is diabetes?

According to the Center for Disease Control[2] (CDC), diabetes is a chronic (long-lasting) health condition that affects how your body turns food into energy. Most of the food you eat is broken down into sugar (glucose) and released into your bloodstream. When your blood sugar goes up, it signals your pancreas to release insulin. Insulin acts like a key to let blood sugar into your body cells for use as energy.

There are three types of diabetes: Type 1, Type 2, and gestational diabetes which occurs during pregnancy.

Type 1 Diabetes

Type 1 Diabetes is thought to be caused by an autoimmune reaction—the body attacking itself by mistake—that stops your body from making insulin. Approximately 5-10% of the people who have diabetes have Type 1. Symptoms of Type 1 often develop quickly. It is usually diagnosed in children, teens, and young adults.

If you have Type 1 Diabetes, you will need to take insulin every day to survive. Currently, no one knows how to prevent Type 1 Diabetes.

Type 2 Diabetes

Type 2 Diabetes means your body does not use insulin well and cannot keep your blood sugar at normal levels. About 90-95% of people with diabetes have Type 2. It develops over many years and is usually diagnosed in adults (but increasing in children, teens, and young adults).

You may not notice any symptoms, so it's important to get your blood sugar tested if you are at risk. Type 2 Diabetes can be prevented or delayed with healthy lifestyle changes such as losing weight, eating healthy, and being active.

Prediabetes

If this information isn't shocking enough, the CDC[3] also reports that in the United States, 88 million adults—more than 1 in 3—have prediabetes. Out of that 88 million, more than 84% of them don't know they have it!

With prediabetes, blood sugar levels are higher than normal, but not high enough to be diagnosed as Type 2 Diabetes. Prediabetes raises your risk for Type 2 Diabetes, heart disease, and stroke. The good news is if you have prediabetes, you can take healthy steps to reverse it.

What are the tools and resources available to help make diabetes better? And if certain types of diabetes are reversible, what can you do right now to manage and possibly reverse diabetes?

---

[2] *Cdc.Gov*,
https://www.cdc.gov/diabetes/basics/diabetes.html.
Accessed 18 May 2021

---

[3] *Cdc.Gov*,
https://www.cdc.gov/diabetes/basics/diabetes.html.
Accessed 18 May 2021.

THE ABCs OF DIABETES

Danielle Batiste

T he time has come again to learn your ABCs. This is especially important in your diabetes health management.

As you read this chapter, you will learn your ABCs and know why it's important to stay on top of your diabetes. I also suggest that you learn how to read your lab results yourself, which provides clarity and for a better conversation with your doctor and health professionals. You can Google this information online, perform research in the library, etc., for guidance on various tests.

For example, I learned that A1C-A is synonymous with A1C. This measurement gives doctors an overall picture of your glucose levels in a three-month period versus what your glucose reading was on the day of the test. This is a true indicator of how well you are managing your diabetes. We will discuss this in more detail shortly.

So, what are the ABCs of diabetes? **A**-(A1C test); **B**-Blood Pressure; and **C**-Cholesterol.

A1C

According to the Mayo Clinic[4], the A1C test is a common blood test used to diagnose Type 1 and Type 2 Diabetes. If you're living

4 "A1C Test." Mayoclinic.Org,
https://www.mayoclinic.org/tests-procedures/a1c-test/about/pac-20384643. Accessed 18 May 2021.

with diabetes, the test is also used to monitor how well you're managing blood sugar levels.

The A1C test is also called the glycated hemoglobin, glycosylated hemoglobin, hemoglobin A1C, or HbA1c test. An A1C test result reflects your average blood sugar level for the past two to three months. Specifically, the A1C test measures what percentage of hemoglobin proteins in your blood are coated with sugar (glycated). Hemoglobin proteins in red blood cells transport oxygen.

The higher your A1C level is, the poorer your blood sugar control and the higher your risk of diabetes complications. So how can you lower your A1C, what do the results mean, and how often should you be tested? Everyday Health offers the following advice[5]:

For some, home blood sugar testing can be an important and useful tool for managing your blood sugar on a day-to-day basis. Still, it only provides a snapshot of what's happening at the moment, not a full picture of what's happened in the long term, says Gregory Dodell MD, assistant clinical professor of medicine, endocrinology, diabetes, and bone disease at Mount Sinai Health System in New York City.

For this reason, your doctor may occasionally administer a blood test that measures your average blood sugar level over the past two to three months. Called the A1C test, or the hemoglobin A1C test,

---

[5] Salomon, Sheryl Huggins, and Kacy Church. "5 Ways to Lower Your A1C." Everydayhealth.Com,

https://www.everydayhealth.com/type-2-
diabetes/treatment/ways- lower-your-a1c/. Accessed 18
May 2021.

this provides another lens on how well your Type 2 Diabetes management plan is working.

If your blood sugar levels have remained stable, the American Diabetes Association (ADA) recommends getting the A1C test two times per year. If your therapy has changed or you are not meeting your glycemic (blood sugar) targets, the ADA recommends getting the test four times per year. This simple blood draw can be done in your doctor's office.

Your A1C score is a valuable part of the diabetes control picture, Dodell says, but it is not the only indicator of your health. Someone who has wide fluctuations in blood sugar levels (which is more common among patients who are taking insulin) may have an A1C at goal because the average over two to three months is good. But the day-to-day fluctuations can lower your quality of life and increase your risk of complications, he cautions.

Diabetes can be a tough condition to manage, Dodell says. He tells his patients to view diabetes management as a job. It takes work, but the time and effort you put into it can result in good control and an improved quality of life. "The key to reaching your A1C goal is trying to follow a healthy lifestyle," he says.

Making these healthy changes can help you improve your day-to- day blood sugar management and lower your A1C:

1. Start an Exercise Plan You Enjoy and Do It Regularly

Find something you enjoy doing that gets your body moving — take your dog for a walk, play a sport with a friend, or ride a stationary bike indoors or a regular bike outdoors.

A good goal is to get 150 minutes of moderate exercise per week, recommends Jordana Turkel, a registered dietitian and certified diabetes educator at Park Avenue Endocrinology and Nutrition in New York City. This is also what the ADA recommends. Different types of exercise (both strength training or resistance training and aerobic exercise) can lower your A1C by making the body more sensitive to insulin, Turkel says. She encourages her patients not to go more than two days in a row without exercising and to aim for two days of strength training.

Be sure to check with your healthcare provider before embarking on an exercise plan, though. He or she can come up with an individualized plan for you.

And if you monitor your blood sugar daily, check it before and after exercise. As the Joslin Diabetes Center at Harvard Medical School explains, exercise can cause your blood sugar to rise—as more is released from the liver—and blood sugar to fall (due to increased insulin sensitivity). Fluctuations in your blood sugar levels can result if you aren't careful. This is

particularly important if you are on insulin or another diabetes medication that causes insulin secretion, such as sulfonylureas, Amaryl (glimepiride), and glinides, such as Prandin (repaglinide) and Starlix (nateglinide).

2. Eat a Balanced Diet with Proper Portion Sizes

It's best to check with a certified diabetes care and education specialist or a registered dietitian-nutritionist to determine what a balanced diet and appropriate portions mean for you. But a great rule of thumb is to visualize your plate for every meal and aim to fill one-half of it with veggies, one-quarter with protein, and one- quarter with whole grains, says Turkel. If you like fruit, limit your portions to a small cup, eaten with a little protein or lean fat to help you digest the fruit carbohydrates in a manner that is less likely to spike your blood sugar level.

Also, avoid processed foods as much as possible, and say no to sugary sodas and fruit juice, which are high in carbs and calories, and thus can lead to spikes in blood sugar and contribute to weight gain, according to the ADA.

3. Stick to a Regular Schedule So You Can More Easily

Follow Your Healthy Diet and Lifestyle

Skipping meals, letting too much time pass between meals, or

eating too much or too often can cause your blood sugar levels

to fall and rise too much, the ADA points out. This is especially true if you are taking insulin or certain diabetes drugs. Your doctor can help you determine the best meal schedule for your lifestyle.

4. Follow the Diabetes Treatment Plan Your Healthcare Team Recommends

Diabetes treatment is very individualized, noted an article published in May 2014 in ***Diabetes Spectrum***. After all, factors including how long you've lived with the disease, your socioeconomic status, and any other conditions you're living with can play a role in the best treatment approach for you.

Your healthcare team will help you determine the steps you need to take to successfully manage diabetes. Always talk to your doctor before making any changes, such as starting a very low- carbohydrate diet, beginning a new exercise regimen, and especially before making any medication or insulin changes.

5. Check Your Blood Sugar Levels as Your Doctor Has Directed

Work with your doctor to determine if, and how often, you should check your blood sugar. You may be tempted to pick up an A1C home testing kit, but Dowdell does not recommend

doing that. As he mentions, day-to-day fluctuations in your blood sugar can be masked by an A1C result that is at your

goal level.

Instead, if you have a personal continuous glucose monitor such as a Dexcom G6 or a Freestyle Libre (or can get one from your healthcare provider), Dowdell recommends checking your "time in range" to see if you are at the optimal level. For many people that is 70 to 180 milligrams per deciliter (mg/dL) (3.9 to 10 mmol/L), according to ADA guidelines. Having your A1C checked by your healthcare provider every three to six months is sufficient, he adds.

Understanding your A1C levels is an important part of your overall diabetes management. If you have any questions about your A1C levels or what they mean, do not hesitate to ask your doctor.

BLOOD PRESSURE

Your blood pressure should be checked at every doctor's appointment. Make sure you speak with your doctor to know your target blood pressure rate. Why?

As John Hopkins Medicine reports[6], high blood pressure is twice as likely to strike a person with diabetes than a person without diabetes. Left untreated, high blood pressure can lead to heart disease and stroke. In fact, a person with diabetes and high blood pressure is four times as likely to develop heart disease than someone who does not have either of the

conditions. About two- thirds of adults with diabetes have blood pressure greater than

130/80 mm Hg or use prescription medications for hypertension.

Blood pressure is the force of the blood pushing against the artery walls. Each time the heart beats, it is pumping blood into these arteries, resulting in the highest blood pressure when the heart contracts and is pumping the blood. High blood pressure, or hypertension, directly increases the risk of coronary heart disease (heart attack) and stroke (brain attack). With high blood pressure, the arteries may have an increased resistance against the flow of blood, causing the heart to pump harder to circulate the blood.

Two numbers are used to measure blood pressure. The

number on the top, the systolic pressure, refers to the pressure inside the artery when the heart contracts and is pumping the blood through the body. The number on the bottom, the diastolic pressure, refers to the pressure inside the artery when the heart is at rest and is filling with blood. Both the systolic and diastolic pressures are recorded as "mm Hg" (millimeters of mercury).

According to the National Heart, Lung, and Blood Institute of the National Institutes of Health (NHLBI), high blood pressure for adults is defined as:

- 140 mm Hg or greater systolic pressure and

90 mm Hg or greater diastolic pressure
- NHLBI guidelines for *prehypertension*

  are:

  - 120 mm Hg – 139 mm Hg systolic pressure and
  - 80 mm Hg – 89 mm Hg diastolic pressure

NHLBI guidelines define normal blood pressure as follows:

- Less than 120 mm Hg systolic pressure and
- Less than 80 mm Hg diastolic pressure

Often, people with high blood pressure do not have noticeable symptoms. If the blood pressure is greatly elevated, a person may experience the following symptoms including (can vary):

- Headache
- Dizziness
- Blurred vision

The symptoms of high blood pressure may resemble other medical conditions or problems. Always consult your doctor for a diagnosis.

The American Diabetes Association recommends the following to help prevent the onset of high blood pressure:

✓ Reduce your salt intake
✓ Engage in stress-relieving activities

✓ Exercise regularly
✓ Get to and stay at a healthy
✓ weight Avoid excessive alcohol intake
✓ Stop smoking and avoid exposure to secondhand
✓ smoke Monitor your blood pressure

6 "Diabetes and High Blood Pressure."
Hopkinsmedicine.Org,
https://www.hopkinsmedicine.org/health/conditions-and-diseases/diabetes/diabetes-and- high-blood-pressure.
Accessed 17 May 2021

CHOLESTEROL

Healthline [7] provides the following information as a guide on diabetes and high cholesterol:

Diabetes and high cholesterol often occur together. If you have both diabetes and high cholesterol, you're not alone. The American Heart Association (AHA) states that diabetes often lowers HDL (good) cholesterol levels and raises triglycerides and LDL (bad) cholesterol levels. Both of these increase the risk for heart disease and stroke.

- An LDL cholesterol level under 100 milligrams/deciliter (mg/dL) is considered ideal.
- 100–129 mg/dL is close to ideal.
- 130–159 mg/dL is borderline elevated.

High cholesterol levels can be dangerous. Cholesterol is a type of fat that can build up inside the arteries. Over time, it can harden to form a stiff plaque, that damages arteries, making them stiff and narrow, inhibiting blood flow. The heart has to work harder to pump blood and the risk for heart attack and stroke goes up.

---

[7] Story, Colleen M. "A Guide to Living with Diabetes and High Cholesterol." Healthline.Com, 17 Apr. 2017,

https://www.healthline.com/health/high-cholesterol/treating-with-statins/guide-to-diabetes-and-high-cholesterol.

Researchers don't have all the answers and continue to grapple with how diabetes and high cholesterol are related. In one study published in The Journal of Lipid Research Trusted Source, they found that blood sugar, insulin, and cholesterol all interact with each other in the body and are affected by each other. They just weren't sure exactly how.

Meanwhile, what's important is that you're aware of the combination between the two. Even if you keep your blood sugar levels under control, your LDL cholesterol levels may still go up. However, you can control both of these conditions with medications and good lifestyle habits. The main goal is to reduce your risk of heart disease and stroke.

The takeaway? Diabetes and high cholesterol can often occur together, but there are ways to manage both conditions. Maintaining a healthy lifestyle and monitoring your cholesterol levels when you have diabetes are important ways of managing both conditions.

DIABETES MADE BETTER

An essential part of managing your diabetes is to be active and proactive. We are in control and need to do what is necessary for optimum health and a better quality of life.

Metformin

Metformin[8] is an oral diabetes medicine that helps control blood sugar levels. It is used together with diet and exercise to improve blood sugar control in adults with Type 2 Diabetes mellitus.

Many diabetics do not like Metformin, but everyone is different. I will tell you that my first seven days on Metformin felt like a mini hell. I had diarrhea and I felt like I was losing everything. The funny thing is my medicine only started working when I arrived for my shift at work. I almost felt like this drug knew my work schedule and wanted to make my life hell.

But after those seven days, I cannot give you one single complaint about Metformin because it has been fine since then. If you are having any issues with this medication or any other medication your

---

[8] "Metformin." Drugs.Com, https://www.drugs.com/metformin.html. Accessed 18 May 2021.

doctor prescribes, do not just stop taking it. Always consult your doctor and be honest.

7 Keys to live, feel, and look good while maintaining your diabetes

1. Drink lots of water

Whether it is from your physician or dietician, you have probably heard the advice to drink lots of water over and over again. Before you tune me out, here are a few facts you might be unaware of, courtesy of Christel Oerum, certified personal trainer, author, diabetes advocate, and founder of Diabetes Strong[9]:

- When you don't drink enough water, the glucose in your bloodstream becomes more concentrated and that leads to higher blood sugar levels. Both mild and severe dehydration can have a notable impact on your diabetes.

- Even a mild level of dehydration — something you may not even feel — could easily leave your blood sugar levels 50 to 100 mg/dL higher than if you were drinking enough water.

---

[9] Oerum, Christel. "Water and Diabetes: Are You Drinking Enough Water?" Diabetesstrong.Com, 15 May

2019, https://diabetesstrong.com/water-diabetes-
drinking- enough-water/.

- If you're consistently dehydrated on a daily basis, you might even be compensating with higher insulin levels than you'd need if your body was getting the water it needed.

- More severe levels of dehydration, on the other hand, can drive blood sugars very high very quickly. For example, repeated vomiting from food poisoning or a stomach virus can lead to very sudden high blood sugar levels. But after an IV of fluids at the emergency room, you'll likely see your blood sugar drop quickly towards normal levels without additional insulin.

- It's the simple issue of severe dehydration causing the glucose in your bloodstream to become extremely concentrated and then quickly diluting it with plenty of fluids.

Now do you feel different about water? So, the next time your doctor or health professional talks about the importance of water, **believe him or her**!

2. Healthy lifestyle changes

Let's talk about "sugars and starch." Most of the American diet is filled with sugary treats, decadent desserts, and starchy foods. There are even hidden sugars in certain food items that are salty or bitter by nature.

Now we all know that no one needs to have a consistent diet of candy bars, sweet treats, and high starch foods. But if you are diabetic, you need to be selective when it comes to your carbohydrate intake. Here's why, courtesy of the American Diabetes Association:[10]

When you eat or drink foods that have carbohydrates—also known as carbs—your body breaks those carbs down into glucose (a type of sugar) which then raises the level of glucose in your blood. Your body uses that glucose for fuel to keep you going throughout the day. This is what you probably know of as your "blood glucose" or "blood sugar." When it comes to managing diabetes, the carbs you eat play an important role. After your body breaks down those carbs into glucose, your pancreas releases insulin to help your cells absorb that glucose.

When someone's blood glucose—or blood sugar—is too high, it is called hyperglycemia. There are a few causes for "highs," including not having enough insulin in your body to process the glucose in the blood or the cells in your body not effectively reacting to the insulin that is released, leaving extra glucose in the blood.

A low blood glucose is known as hypoglycemia. "Lows" can sometimes be caused by not consuming enough carbohydrates or an imbalance in medications. In short, the

------

[10] "Understanding Carbs." Diabetes.Org, https://www.diabetes.org/nutrition/understanding-carbs. Accessed 16 May 2021.

carbs we consume impact our blood sugar—so balance is key!

There are three main types of carbohydrates in food—starches, sugar, and fiber. As you'll see on the nutrition labels for the food you buy, the term "total carbohydrate" refers to all three of these types. The goal is to choose carbs that are nutrient-dense, which means they are rich in fiber, vitamins, and minerals and low in added sugars, sodium, and unhealthy fats.

For the record, this advice isn't just for diabetics but applies also to those who have trouble losing weight. Have you heard the phrase "insulin resistance?" The Obesity Medicine Association[11] defines insulin resistance and what can be done about it:

Insulin resistance happens when the body's cells become resistant to insulin and ever-increasing amounts of it are required to have the same "unlocking" effect on body cells. Insulin resistance is a precursor to prediabetes and Type 2 Diabetes.

Insulin resistance can happen due to a combination of genetics and lifestyle leading to an inflammatory process in the body.

---

[11] "Obesity and Insulin Resistance." Obesitymedicine.Org, 24 Aug. 2018, https://obesitymedicine.org/obesity-and-insulin-resistance/.

There are many biological stress factors that can set insulin resistance in motion including excess nutrition.

When this happens, the body struggles to maintain blood sugar at the correct level. In an effort to keep blood sugar in the normal range, more insulin is secreted from beta cells in the pancreas. A veritable tug-of-war ensues between forces attempting to remove and store sugar in the body's cells and those cells themselves that are "full" and becoming less sensitive to the actions of insulin. At some point, tests for fasting blood sugar, postprandial blood sugars (blood sugar checked after a meal), and/or HgbA1c will start to increase. Elevated triglycerides, as well as LDL-C (bad cholesterol), may also be seen.

Insulin resistance is uncommonly identified prior to the onset of prediabetes or Type 2 Diabetes, as most patients do not have symptoms. However, there are certain signs or risk factors that can alert you to the increased likelihood of insulin resistance, such as increased waist circumference, weight gain predominantly in the abdominal region, and rising triglycerides and LDL-C (bad cholesterol).

There are a number of ways to improve one's sensitivity to insulin, thereby helping to break the cycle of ever-increasing insulin levels:

- Work on decreasing chronic stress

- Get a good night's sleep

- Avoid sugar-sweetened beverages and added sugars

- Moderate your processed carbohydrate intake (all carbohydrates are NOT created equal!)

- Move or get NEAT (non-exercise activity time)

Many studies now show that decreasing chronic stress can decrease cortisol hormone levels thereby lowering blood sugar. A good night's sleep not only leaves you with more energy for NEAT but also decreases the hunger hormone ghrelin, so you feel less of an inclination to eat. Movement sensitizes muscle to insulin thereby decreasing insulin resistance. Finally, taking care to limit processed foods lessens blood sugar and insulin spikes that can occur with sugar-sweetened beverages and sugars added to foods.

3. Cut Back on Alcohol

At this point, you understand the importance of making wise decisions in what you consume in food and beverage. However, there are special considerations for diabetics when it comes to alcohol consumption including its interference with your medication and particular diabetes type. Some would advise you to do "all things in moderation," but the best advice is to consult your doctor to see if alcohol consumption is recommended for you and, if so, in what proportion. WebMD[12] provides the following advice:

If you have diabetes, drinking alcohol may cause your blood sugar to either rise or fall. Plus, alcohol has a lot of calories.

If you drink, do it occasionally and only when your diabetes and blood sugar levels are well-controlled. If you are following a calorie-controlled meal plan, one drink of alcohol should be counted as two fat exchanges. Learn more about the effects of alcohol on diabetes.

4. Eat a Well-Balanced Diet

We discussed this in Tip #2, but there are a few bonus things I want to share. I use a portion plate to make sure I eat in balance and eat the things I need. It is easy to forget and just pile your plate with what pleases your eye and include "some of the things" your body needs. But a balanced diet is the cornerstone of health.

Women, like men, should enjoy a variety of healthy foods from all of the food groups including whole grains, fruits, vegetables, healthy fats, low-fat or fat-free dairy, and lean protein. Your plate

---

[12] Webmd.Com, https://www.webmd.com/diabetes/guide/drinking-alcohol. Accessed 16 May 2021.

and dietary choices should be colorful. Often, unhealthy choices are not.

Again, consult your doctor and health professionals for the ideal meal plan and your special dietary needs. We've got this!

5. Take medication as prescribed

There is not much I am going to say about this except this is not optional. The worst thing you can do to treat your diabetes is to self-medicate.

There is a reason why medicine is prescribed by a medical professional. Yes, I encourage you to continually educate yourself on medications, treatments, and alternatives that are available, but use what you learn to consult with medical professionals.

If you experience side effects, make sure you consult with your doctor first, not reduce or stop taking your medication. Our bodies are different and things can change based on age, diet, and the length of time you have been on your medication. Also, other medications can interact with a new medication and cause certain side effects as well.

Talk to your doctor at all times including when you have major lifestyle changes, are considering major lifestyle changes, or experience any undesirable side effects. It might be as simple as your doctor changing your dosage or prescribing a different medication.

6. Good sleep

Yes, good sleep is vital to everyone's overall health, diabetic or not. I could write an entire book on good sleep, but here is why it matters in reference to diabetes and blood sugar management according to the Sleep Foundation[13]:

> Just as diabetes can cause sleep problems, sleep problems also appear to play a role in diabetes. Getting poor sleep or less restorative slow-wave sleep has been linked to high blood sugar levels in people with diabetes and prediabetes. However, it's not entirely clear whether one causes the other or whether more variables are at work. Researchers believe that sleep restriction may affect blood sugar levels due to its effects on insulin, cortisol, and oxidative stress.
>
> One-quarter of people with diabetes report sleeping less than six hours or more than eight hours a night, which puts them at a higher risk of having elevated blood sugar. In addition to raising blood sugar levels in people who already have diabetes, sleep deprivation also raises the risk of developing insulin resistance in the first place. This link becomes apparent as early as childhood.

---

[13] "Diabetes and Sleep: Sleep Disturbances & Coping." Sleepfoundation.Org, 20 Nov. 2020, https://www.sleepfoundation.org/physical-health/lack-of-sleep-and-diabetes.

Sleep deprivation raises levels of ghrelin, the hunger hormone, and decreases levels of leptin, the hormone that makes us feel full. To compensate for lower energy levels, people who sleep poorly may be more likely to seek relief in foods that raise blood sugar and put them at risk of obesity, which is a risk factor for diabetes.

In addition to its immediate effects on blood sugar levels, poor sleep can take a long-term toll on individuals with Type2 Diabetes. Those who resort to sleep medication or who have trouble staying asleep are more likely to report feeling serious psychological distress. There is also tentative evidence to suggest that people with diabetes who do not get enough sleep may be at a higher risk for cognitive decline later in life.

Lack of quality, restorative sleep is no laughing matter. Take every effort you can to get enough sleep and quality sleep. Turn off your electronic devices an hour before your bedtime and make sure you stop eating a few hours before. You may also stop drinking a few hours before bedtime to reduce the frequency of your bedroom trips throughout the night. Talk to your medical professional if you are having problems sleeping which may be an indication of other disorders or health issues.

7. **Protect your skin**

Diabetes can wreak havoc on your skin and can cause bacterial or fungal infections. Check your body for skin concerns daily, especially in skin folds such as underarms, between your toes, and the groin area. Help protect your skin by keeping it clean and dry at all times.

If you notice an injury, even a minor cut, clean it with soap and water. Talk to your doctor if you notice serious injuries to your skin or have a condition you cannot treat on your own. I do a skin check every day and I take my own supplies when going for pedicures to make sure they focus directly on my feet. Your medical professional can give you the appropriate guidelines to follow for diabetic manicures and pedicures.

Are you connecting the dots?

Remember, I told you at the beginning of this book that when I was first diagnosed, I was in denial. I ignored all the above advice and did what I wanted until I no longer could. The truth is I got sick and tired of being sick and tired and, if you're reading this book, you are probably in the same boat.

The facts are the facts and we all have a choice. Diabetes does not have to be a death sentence and we are not powerless victims of this disease. Every day we can make choices to live our best lives by controlling our health through fitness, diet, and mindset. **We can eat and drink our health or eat and drink our death.** We can use movement through exercise and fitness to restore our energy, vitality, and youthfulness or we can be couch potatoes of inflammation, fat, tiredness, pain, and numbness. But either choice is ours, day by day and minute by minute. **What will you choose today: life or death?**

Lastly, build social support. Your social support can be life-changing and lifesaving. While diabetes is an individual disease, it not only affects your life but the lives of those around you. You will need help in this journey and others can aid you when necessary but they must know how to help or support you. For example, what if your blood sugar drops and you experience hypoglycemia? Your social support should be aware of your needs like your medication intake or how frequently you need to eat. If they have to call 911, they should be able to tell them what type of diabetes you have, when was the last time you ate, and the symptoms you're experiencing. Their actions, timeliness, and the information they provide to medical professionals can make the difference between life and death.

MY JOURNEY FROM DIAGNOSIS
TO NOW

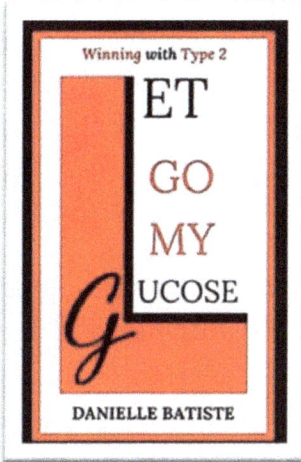

This is my FAVORITE book in the world. Why? Well, I wrote it!

Seriously, the book goes into my first years of living with diabetes and my ignorance of it because I still did not quite understand this disease, but I did notice changes in me and my body.

In this chapter, I want to be very transparent with you about what diabetes is and what it can do to our bodies if we do not take the steps to keep it under control.

Let Go of My Glucose is my second book. I wrote this after finding out in June of 2013 that I was a Type 2 diabetic.

To be honest with you, I did not believe it because, in my mind, the only people who get diabetes were old and fat and I was neither, so I thought my doctor was pulling my leg. This began my journey of denial and that is where I stayed for one year and some months until I had my first symptoms.

Now, mind you, I did go to all the classes that my doctor had set up for me, so that is how I knew what the symptoms of diabetes were. After that jolt of reality, I came to my senses and started reading everything I could on Type 2 Diabetes. So, in this book, I am very transparent on everything that has and will continue to happen to me as I go along this journey because diabetes is not something we can cure or think we are better than. However, what we can do is read, live better, adopt a healthier lifestyle, and stay active.

Let us not get behind it. To stay ahead of it, we need determination, dedication, and mindset. If your mind is not right, your body will not follow.

How Diabetes Affected My Body

When I was first diagnosed with diabetes in June 2013, I did not believe it, so I would not follow directions. Please do not take that route. Listen to your doctor and handle the situation head-on. Let me tell you how diabetes affected my body.

When you travel with diabetes, you must be vigilant in your travels. Packing isn't like what you are used to, so you must think about your body, how long of a trip this will be, and what needs to be at your fingertips for this trip.

The first thing I do when I plan my trip is let the airlines know I'm a diabetic so they are informed that there is someone with medical problems on the plane. I also take my sugar before I leave to make sure it is good, so if it drops I know what it was before boarding and have it written down for emergencies. Sometimes, if the flight is four or more hours, this can trigger my glucose levels to drop, but this is where your preparedness comes into play.

I make sure to have my glucose tablets handy and something to eat that goes straight to the blood like raisins or peanut butter. You don't have to take it all at the same time, but it's good to have it with you. Soda helps too, but I find that the above is a much faster relief for me. Everybody is different, so take that into consideration. Your sugar can drop so fast, and symptoms can occur so lightly at first, that you wouldn't even notice until you start shaking uncontrollably.

Another thing I noticed with my body is that after the trip is over, I feel and look fine, but after I get home and settle, that's when the feeling of sleep overwhelms me. I don't know how to fight that, but that is my body's way of telling me that the trip was too much, even though I seemed fine. One flight was four hours and all I could do when I got home was collapse on the bed. I could not move for about two days before I regained total energy because my body was beat. You would think it was jet lag, at least that's what it felt like, but trust me it is not. It feels like the body has no willpower to move at all, not even to go to the bathroom. It is so tiring that you don't want to eat, but you know you must regain your energy as well. This is extreme fatigue.

Exercising also affects your body if you don't listen to it. The doctor
tells you to exercise three times a week for at least 30 minutes a day, which is good for a diabetic, but not me. I tried to do it at least three to four times a week for about an hour, and my body can usually take it, but my advice is don't do what your body can't handle, only what it can. I also drink a Gatorade

an hour before a workout for the carbs because you will work those carbs back off and it helps keep everything at bay for me. Sometimes I can get away without doing it, but my body will tell me when enough exercising is enough and that I must slow down.

Foods that I did not eat were green vegetables. The only thing green I ate coming from Louisiana—yes, I'm a Louisiana girl—was cabbage. When I became a diabetic, all I kept hearing about was green vegetables. I was so sick of hearing it! The only way I would tolerate eating them was in a smoothie, but eventually, I knew that I had to venture out and taste them. So my husband started me out with broccoli and, the way he sautéed and seasoned them, I fell in love. Broccoli became my first love for green things.

Now peas were another story. Those little things remind me of ticks. I hate to say it but I'm being honest. I don't like peas, I just tolerate them. I love and would eat asparagus all day if I could and, I must say that greens are good for us.

Water has been a great source of love for me as a diabetic and it helps keep me hydrated. I was never one to drink water and it took a long time for people to beat this one into my head. Once I started drinking water and reading different things, I started drinking half of my body weight in ounces. Water cleanses me out better than any colon cleanser or similar product. Water is doing the trick for me and is keeping me regular with everything under control, especially if my sugar goes too high. There's not much I can do when this happens and it serves as my warning sign. If I end up getting a very bad headache, I know my sugar is high. When that happens, I drink a lot of water and flush as much of that poison, or sugar, I possibly can and it usually helps.

I'm not saying that water is the cure-all, but it does work for my body. Water doesn't stop my headache, but it helps.

All I do when my headaches occur is lay down, rest, and let my body do its job.

I was taken off my medicine in April 2017, believe it or not, and I was scared because I had been telling my doctor when my A1C was high, even when it was in the six range, that I wanted to be taken off my medication. When the time came and I was taken off, I was one scared cookie.

She was like, "Now that I'm taking you off, big shot, you have the nerve to be scared?" I said yes, but she took me off anyway, advising me to just try it. Of course, I did.

Now it took a few days because, since my diabetes diagnosis, I became in tune with my body. Remember, I noticed right off the back that Metformin was blocking my sugar cravings (or at least that was what was in my head). I now know what people on alcohol and drugs feel like when they are fiending for something. I see how hard it is to fight these cravings, but you must have strong willpower. Trust me, I lost the fight in the beginning, but I put my mind over matter and refused to let cravings destroy my challenging work. It did for a minute because my A1C went back up to 6.2, which my doctor said was still good, but not good enough for me because I was at four. I worked my butt off to get back there and win the battle.

September 13, 2017, was not a good day for me and this is another reason we diabetics must watch our stress levels when things happen. My grandmother was admitted into the hospital for dehydration but, at the time, I did not know that the diagnosis was dehydration. My grandmother and I are very close and if anything happens to her, I would die.

So, of course, when I got the call that she was in the hospital, I became scared, nervous, and helpless. I didn't think about myself. We tend to forget we have diabetes and all that goes out the window.

For the entire day, I tried to follow the same routine, which was work and my evening kickboxing class. While there, I took my phone with me and I was constantly leaving the floor to go to the back and check to make sure I was not missing a call or text from my sister regarding our grandmother's prognosis. My friend noticed what was going on and finally came to the back with me. I could not text because I was not concentrating on myself and I did not notice that my sugar had dropped to a very low point. I was trying to text but my fingers were shaking so bad that I couldn't hold the phone or text a message. I was unable to form my words properly because I was so out of it and my concentration was completely off. I didn't know what the hell I was saying or thinking.

My friend quickly went out to my car and got the glucose tablet that quickly goes to my bloodstream and gets me back on track. Please be aware of your body when you are going through a stressful situation because your sugar can drop quickly. It only takes seconds for you to be in trouble.

I'm still learning this disease, and you will too, because every day, every week, and every month, there is something new with diabetes. I noticed drier skin, so I had to go to the doctor to get prescription lotion, which helped a little bit. I also noticed a bruise on my back, which was not there before. Please pay attention to your body as well.

When I was younger, I didn't see anything but, trust me, as time goes on things change. Always remember when you get out of the shower to dry in between your toes because that is a dark, moist place that bacteria love to live in. This is a good rule of thumb for everyone, not only diabetics. Do not put lotion between your toes either as it creates a type of moisture that is not good for skin in between there.

When I go to get a pedicure, I don't have my cuticles cut all the time. When I do, I make sure her undivided attention is on my feet so that she does not cut me. With diabetes, you must be sure you are cautious of practically everything you do to make sure you do not get any cuts from anything because it will take a while to heal and you must watch it. If it's taking too long, you must make an appointment with your primary care doctor.

Another thing I noticed with my body is that it does not do well in extreme heat. Being in heat takes all my energy and I'm worn out completely. It makes me feel like I just ran track five times: terrible and all out of sorts.

When I was younger, it would take about 30 minutes to get my energy back, but now that I am older, it takes darn near a day or two for me to feel 100%. So there are changes from my first diagnosis to now.

As a diabetic, I'm very conscious of my weight since I can put it on real fast. Extra weight can be bad for me as it will have my glucose out of control, which would cause my A1C to fluctuate. This can also cause complications with your heart, kidneys, and make things hard to keep under control. Therefore, I exercise at least three to four times a week. I'm not saying you must, but please be conscious of your body and weight too.

As far as a sign that something is wrong, I think it can vary from person to person. I get shaky and that's easily handled with a glucose tablet. My symptom is small, but I do notice.

My doctor asks me about tingling in my toes and blurred vision which, thankfully, I don't get often, but one thing to be aware of: your body is prone to yeast infections (or UTIs) because a diabetic's PH balance is constantly irregular. That's how you go from never having anything to having to adjust to what I called a foreign substance invading your body that you must fight against every day.

In November 2017, I went to the doctor thinking I had a UTI or something. I never had one in my life due to my sugar/glucose acting up, but thank God it wasn't one. However, that's just an example of how I become aware of things my body was doing when things seemed out of whack. If you let it go or ignore it then it will take longer to heal and make the fight that much harder.

On Saturday, December 2nd, 2017, my energy level was beyond high. It was through the roof! I went outside to rake our front and back yard full of leaves. I worked nonstop, only taking mini-breaks occasionally. Our backyard is huge and I raked all the leaves into piles to bag.

My son and husband helped while also cleaning the roof and gutters. I went inside and finished some things and then went out to eat. The whole day was a "10" for me. Then Sunday came and the day was a "2." I was done.

I could barely move, did not want to get up, or eat. This is a classic way of showing how this disease works sometimes where you have good days and bad days.

Having Type 2 Diabetes, you figure you can read this and learn, but when I learned of my diagnosis, I only found half of the personal stuff I'm telling you in the literature I read. I found a lot of material that just touched the surface but I am going to share everything with you from the top to the bottom.

I remember sitting at work with a special pair of shoes trying to be cute. I know I cannot keep them on for more than an hour, so I showed everyone my shoes and then put on flats. Shoes that are made like "witch shoes," (the ones that are pointy), are not good for diabetics because they bunch the toes up, are painful, and cause corns we cannot afford to get because of the long healing process. If that happens or you have any foot issues, please consult with a podiatric doctor. All foot problems need to be taken care of as soon as possible to avoid amputation.

Regardless of what is going on in my life, I must watch what I eat, exercise, and be vigilant. Being diabetic does not mean that I'm not human. I get emotional, cry and holler, "Why me?" There are days when it gets tiring and grinds my nerves. Some days, I wish I could just be free enough to feel like me without diabetes and the steps necessary to manage it. Reality eventually sinks back in, though.

We will have our ups and downs. We're not perfect, but we have to keep going and keep on living. We can't let diabetes get us down all the time.

My Biggest Challenges and Rewards

My biggest challenges with diabetes are counting my carbs and watching what I ate. I was so used to eating what I wanted, but a lifestyle change is big and drastic. Going to the grocery store and trying to buy things you never ate before, is time-consuming and expensive so you almost want to revert to your old ways of eating and say *forget this*. Going backward is so much easier than going forward to a new and healthier you.

Let's talk about taking these drugs and medication: Metformin with Glyburide. I had to take these twice a day: one for breakfast and one for dinner. The one for breakfast was the worst because it was around the time I had to go to work and the first seven days of it gave me diarrhea. Diarrhea is never good, but especially not when you must get on the road and go to work. Eventually, the misery was over.

I must admit that the first year was hard for me because I was in denial about having the disease. The symptoms did not manifest themselves all at once, so I remained skeptical about my condition. I soon learned the shakiness of my hands was when my sugar was high. I would get migraine-type headaches and all I could do was lay down and regroup.

Another thing diabetes does is drain your energy. When I say drain your energy, I mean going from ten to zero and sometimes it would take me three to four hours to regain my stamina. One time, it took an entire day for me to get myself together.

Diabetes is no joke and I found that out the hard way. On top of the lifestyle change, you need regular, once-a-year diabetic eye exams to make sure nothing changes with your vision. Keep your feet healthy and dry, especially between your toes (no lotion there at all)

Once my kickboxing classes started, the road began. Between walking and kickboxing, my body transformed into a fighting machine that diabetes could not mess with and I took charge of myself and my life. My A1C and everything else started coming down, but it didn't happen overnight. I fought for the body I'm in now and I must fight to continue to stay in it.

I was never a water drinker, but I now drink it faithfully and that has helped my body flush out a lot of toxins. At my last doctor's appointment, I came out with the best news of my life. After all of my challenging work, determination, and sacrifices (despite being hard-headed in the beginning), my sugar and cholesterol (good and bad), were great. My A1C was 4.8 (yes)!

When my A1C was 6.2 and 5.2, I kept asking my doctor about taking me off the medicine and she said no. When I finally got to 4.8, I was afraid to mention it. She reminded me that I had been asking to come off the medication and now I was a little scared, but she took me off anyway.

I still have to go for regular follow-up exams. The doctor told me my Type 2 Diabetes disease is controlled with diet and exercise. It's called determination and not letting diabetes beat you – you beat diabetes!

_____
_____

WHEN GOING TO THE DOCTOR

J ust something to remember to take with you when going to the doctor. Always bring your most recent two weeks of blood sugar readings and this form to your next visit:

Eye doctor's name / Date of most recent examination

_____ | __/__

Heart doctor's name / Most recent visit

_____ | __/__

Foot doctor's name / Most recent visit
Diabetes specialist's name / Most recent visit

_____ | __/__

Current Medications (Name, dose, time taken)

_____ | __/__

_____ | __/__

Current Medications (Name, dose, time taken) cont.

_____ | __/___

_____ | __/___

_____ | __/___

_____ | __/___

_____ | __/___

How often do you test your blood sugar? (circle answer)

Rarely

When I feel bad

1 or 2 times a

week Daily

2 times daily

4 times daily

What time do you usually test your blood sugar (circle all that apply)?

Fasting

After

breakfast

Before Lunch

After Lunch

Before Supper

After Supper

Before

bedtime

How many times in the last week have you had low blood sugar? _

How many times in the last month? ____

What time of day does your low blood sugar occur? _

_____

AM/PM

How do you treat low blood sugar episodes (circle all that apply)?

Glucose tablets

Juice

Fruit

Other _____

If you are using insulin, do you have a Glucagon kit?

Yes/No

I also want to let you know about the glycemic index. I personally don't hear a lot of diabetics talking about it, so I wanted to because it's very useful to us. I first learned about it while doing my research and found it to be very helpful in the food we choose to eat to work in harmony with our diabetes.

According to the Harvard Publishing Health of Harvard Medical School [14] , measuring carbohydrate effects can help glucose management:

---

[14] "Glycemic Index for 60+ Foods." Harvard.Edu, 3 Feb. 2015, https://www.health.harvard.edu/diseases-and-conditions/glycemic-index-and-glycemic- load-for-100-foods.

The glycemic index is a value assigned to foods based on how slowly or how quickly those foods cause increases in blood glucose levels. Foods low on the glycemic index (GI) scale tend to release glucose slowly and steadily. Foods high on the glycemic index release glucose rapidly.

Low GI foods tend to foster weight loss, while foods high on the GI scale help with energy recovery after exercise, or to offset hypo- (or insufficient) glycemia. Long-distance runners would tend to favor foods high on the glycemic index, while people with pre-or full-blown diabetes would need to concentrate on low GI foods. Why?

People with Type 1 diabetes can't produce sufficient quantities of insulin and those with Type 2 diabetes are resistant to insulin. With both types of diabetes, faster glucose release from high GI foods leads to spikes in blood sugar levels. The slow and steady release of glucose in low-glycemic foods helps maintain good glucose control.

To help you understand how the foods you are eating might impact your blood glucose level, here is an abbreviated chart of the glycemic index for more than 60 common foods:

FOOD	Glycemic index (glucose = 100)
HIGH-CARBOHYDRATE FOODS	
White wheat bread*	75 ± 2
Whole wheat/whole meal bread	74 ± 2
Specialty grain bread	
Unleavened wheat bread	70 ± 5
Wheat roti	62 ± 3
Chapatti	52 ± 4
Corn tortilla	46 ± 4
White rice, boiled*	73 ± 4
Brown rice, boiled	68 ± 4
Barley	28 ± 2
Sweet corn	52 ± 5
Spaghetti, white	49 ± 2
Spaghetti, whole meal	48 ± 5
Rice noodles†	53 ± 7
Udon noodles	55 ± 7

FOOD	Glycemic index (glucose = 100)
Couscous†	65 ± 4

BREAKFAST CEREALS	
FOOD	Glycemic index (glucose = 100)
Cornflakes	81 ± 6
Wheat flake biscuits	69 ± 2
Porridge, rolled oats	55 ± 2
Instant oat porridge	79 ± 3
Rice porridge/congee	78 ± 9
Millet porridge	67 ± 5
Muesli	57 ± 2
FRUIT AND FRUIT PRODUCTS	
Apple, raw†	36 ± 2
Orange, raw†	43 ± 3

Banana, raw†	51 ± 3

FOOD	Glycemic index (glucose = 100)
FRUIT AND FRUIT PRODUCTS	
Pineapple, raw	59 ± 8
Mango, raw†	51 ± 5
Watermelon, raw	76 ± 4
Dates, raw	42 ± 4
Peaches, canned†	43 ± 5
Strawberry jam/jelly	49 ± 3
Apple juice	41 ± 2
Orange juice	50 ± 2
VEGETABLES	
Potato, boiled	78 ± 4
Potato, instant mash	87 ± 3
Potato, French fries	63 ± 5
Carrots, boiled	39 ± 4
Sweet potato, boiled	63 ± 6

FOOD	Glycemic index (glucose = 100)
VEGETABLES	
Pumpkin, boiled	64 ± 7
Plantain/green banana	55 ± 6
Taro, boiled	53 ± 2
Vegetable soup	48 ± 5
DAIRY PRODUCTS AND ALTERNATIVES	
Milk, full fat	39 ± 3
Milk, skim	37 ± 4
Ice cream	51 ± 3
Yogurt, fruit	41 ± 2
Soy milk	34 ± 4
Rice milk	86 ± 7

FOOD	Glycemic index (glucose = 100)
LEGUMES	
Chickpeas	28 ± 9
Kidney beans	24 ± 4
Lentils	32 ± 5
Soya beans	16 ± 1
SNACK PRODUCTS	
Chocolate	40 ± 3
Popcorn	65 ± 5
Potato crisps	56 ± 3
Soft drink/soda	59 ± 3
Rice crackers/crisps	87 ± 2

FOOD	Glycemic index (glucose = 100)
SUGARS	
Fructose	15 ± 4
Sucrose	65 ± 4
Glucose	103 ± 3
Honey	61 ± 3

Data are means ± SEM.

* Low-GI varieties were also identified.

† Average of all available data.

TRAVELING WITH DIABETES:
THE TO-DO-LIST

B efore I share the stories of two others who are conquering diabetes, I want to leave you with a to-do list to make traveling as a diabetic easier. If you ever experience hypoglycemia while on a plane, it will make you feel so bad that you will be screaming to get off! Let me empower you and save you the embarrassment.

When traveling, pack all essentials such as:

- Medication/insulin

- Needles

- Alcohol pads

- Freestyle Libre (make sure you have extra sensors) or Accu- Check (if still used, or both)

- Any fast-acting carbs (for hypoglycemia), at least 15 grams. I prefer to travel with glucose tablets or liquid glucose drinks.

Before you go on your trip, please learn the area you will be staying at because you need to know the closest hospital and drugstore in case of emergencies. Also, if you can get a medical bracelet, the most important thing to look up is the time zone because that plays a big part in your diabetes. It can knock you out of whack. For flights, I normally pack my meal in case my glucose goes down.

Before You Go:

1. Visit your doctor for a checkup to ensure you're fit for the trip.
Make sure to ask your doctor:

- How your planned activities could affect your diabetes and what to do about it.

- How to adjust your insulin doses if you're traveling to a
different time zone.

- To provide prescriptions for your medicines in case you lose them or run out.

- If you'll need any vaccines.

- To write a letter stating that you have diabetes and why you need your medical supplies.

2. Just in case, locate pharmacies and clinics close to where you're
staying.

3. Get a medical ID bracelet that states you have diabetes and any other health conditions.

4. Get travel insurance in case you miss your flight or need medical care.

5. Order a special meal for the flight that fits with your meal plan or pack your own.

6. Packing:

- Put your diabetes supplies in a carry-on bag (insulin could get too cold in your checked luggage). Think about bringing a smaller bag to have at your seat for insulin, glucose tablets, and snacks.

- Pack twice as much medicine as you think you'll need. Carry medicines in the pharmacy bottles they came in or ask your pharmacist to print out extra labels you can attach to plastic bags.

- Be sure to pack healthy snacks like fruit, raw veggies, and nuts.

7. Airport security:

- Get an optional TSA notification card to help the screening process go more quickly and smoothly.

- Good news: people with diabetes are exempt from the 3.4 oz. liquid rule for medicines, fast-acting carbs like juice, and gel packs to keep insulin cool.

- A continuous glucose monitor or insulin pump could be damaged going through the X-ray machine. You don't have to disconnect from either; ask for a hand inspection instead.

8. Visit CDC's Travelers' Health site for more helpful resources.

Don't leave home without:

- Doctor's letter and prescriptions

- Snacks and glucose tablets

- Extra insulin and diabetes medicines

While You're Traveling

9. If you're driving, pack a cooler with healthy foods and plenty of water to drink.

10. Don't store insulin or diabetes medicine in direct sunlight or a hot car; keep them in the cooler too. Don't put insulin directly on ice or a gel pack.

11. Heat can also damage your blood sugar monitor, insulin pump, and other diabetes equipment. Don't leave them in a hot car, by a pool, in direct sunlight, or on the beach. The same goes for supplies such as test strips.

12. You can find healthy food options at the airport or a roadside restaurant:

- Fruit, nuts, sandwiches, yogurt

- Salads with chicken or fish (skip the dried fruit and croutons)

- Eggs and omelets

- Burgers with a lettuce wrap instead of a bun

- Fajitas (skip the tortillas and rice)

Say goodbye to worry when you pack your diabetes supplies in a carry-on bag:

13. Stop and get out of the car or walk up and down the aisle of the plane or train every hour or two to prevent blood clots (people with diabetes are at higher risk).

14. Set an alarm on your phone to take medicine if you're traveling
across time zones.

Once You're There:

15. Your blood sugar may be out of your target range at first, but your body should adjust in a few days. Check your blood sugar often and treat highs or lows as instructed by your doctor or diabetes educator.

16. If you're going to be more active than usual, check your blood sugar before and after and make adjustments to food, activity, and insulin as needed.

17. Food is a huge highlight (and temptation!) on a cruise. Avoid the giant buffet, and order off the spa menu (healthier choices), low-carb menu (most ships have one), or order something tasty that fits in your meal plan from the 24-hour room service instead.

18. Don't overdo physical activity during the heat of the day. Avoid getting a sunburn and don't go barefoot, not even on the beach.

19. High temperatures can change how your body uses insulin. You may need to test your blood sugar more often and adjust your insulin dose and what you eat and drink.

20. You may not be able to find everything you need to manage your diabetes away from home, especially in another country. Learn some useful phrases, such as "I have diabetes" and "Where is the nearest pharmacy?"

21. If your vacation is in the great outdoors, bring wet

wipes so you can clean your hands before you check your blood sugar.

How to take extra care of yourself during a trip:

When your schedule changes, it's more difficult to predict and account for blood sugar shifts. Throw in a host of new activities or much more downtime than usual, and you'll likely have to make some careful changes to prevent a diabetic emergency.

Estimate carbs and calories before meals:

It's a good idea to look up some of the foods you expect to be eating on an online calorie-counting website to see how many carbs and calories they contain.

Check your blood glucose levels more often:

When mealtimes tend to shift and you're eating out more than you usually do, you'll probably need to check your blood glucose more often to stay on track. Aim to test your blood before and after you eat a meal for the first time to see how it affects your body.

Be kind to your body:

- While you're out exploring the world, remember that long days of sightseeing can drain your glucose levels and lazy afternoons by the pool can lead to higher blood glucose levels.

- If you are enjoying a different level of activity than you usually do, be prepared to test your blood sugar more often throughout the day.

- It's not always easy to continue your regular lifestyle, especially when you're traveling through different time zones. Still, it's important not to stray too far from your usual routine.

- You may be flexible when it comes to new activities, cuisines, and schedules, but your diabetes is not as flexible. Still, with some planning, you'll be able to keep exploring the world.

MY DIABETES JOURNEY
CHANGED MY LIFE
DAVID NELSON

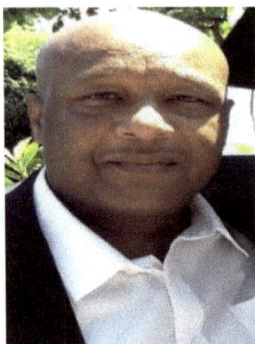

I remember the day I was told that I had diabetes. It was like someone had just told me my nose was running and here's a napkin: it didn't mean anything to me. I was nonchalant, not knowing I was in for the ride of my life.

The effects and signs of diabetes started way before my diagnosis from my doctor. I was, as I later found out, the typical hard-nosed black male that didn't believe in doctors. My baby, who would turn out to be my wife and the mother of my children, noticed I was running around with all sorts of energy and would then suddenly crash like a dope fiend junkie. Then the bouts of suddenly passing out started.

I could merely be walking through the house and then notice I was on the floor, not remembering going down or anything. I'd be walking behind Nakita while looking at the back of her and suddenly be staring from ground height at her feet. These events, along with others, are what led me to my first adult doctor visit.

I fought every adjustment the doctor required of me. From the medications to the life changes, I just brushed it all off as though it would go away just like everything else. After five years of dealing with diabetes, a light bulb went off in my head.

My wife, who most men would describe as hard-nosed, was on me day in and day out about taking diabetes seriously, but to no avail. I didn't listen until a new symptom struck me. My legs started swelling up with fluid and that made me want to learn about what was happening to me, but I was still not as serious as I should have been but at least I was listening.

I went to see a Nephrologist and I was told the combination of years of neglect of my body, my poor management of my diabetes coupled with my Metformin use, were affecting my kidneys. My legs would swell like a balloon with constant pain and headaches.

I continued working, which kept me away from my wife's eyesight. She would call, constantly checking on my health. I always told her that everything was good, but truthfully, I was suffering and my health was declining.

I would get off work and all I could do was bathe and lay down because my legs would be so swollen and in pain that it would take me being off my feet until the next day for the swelling to reduce and for me to feel normal. This went on for months until my job was over.

When I came home and walked through the door, the look on my wife's face was a look I would never forget. She said to me, "No more will I ever let you out of my sight." Those were her first words to me.

Over the next few years together, she worked me back to health, changing our eating habits, and vowed that she would make a family change by keeping everyone healthy while nurturing me back to health. We created a gym within our home, working out every other day, and walked on the treadmill every day with regular A1C and blood pressure checks.

I learned a few diabetes tricks like taking a spoonful of mustard when my sugar levels were up or when my sugar would drop to break a glucose tablet in half by chewing and swallowing one half and letting the other half dissolve slowly in my mouth. Chewing would immediately stop it from dropping and the slow dissipation would slowly bring my sugar up, not putting too much strain on my heart.

To control my cholesterol levels, I would take a teaspoon of Virgin organic olive oil in the morning before I ate or drunk anything and a teaspoon at bedtime. When it was time to see my doctor, they would ask me about my pill arrangement and I would tell them what they wanted to hear and that was that.

For example, I told them I was taking my cholesterol and other meds, and they would tell me it's because of my regiment, but I knew my cholesterol was under control from olive oil. I had never taken a cholesterol pill in my life and my A1C was at level. I was doing good, but as faith would have it, all those years of neglect had taken their toll on my kidneys. I was put on dialysis and, as true to the person she is, she sat me down and said to me: "I won't let you let this cripple you or make you a slave to it."

She took me to the dialysis clinic and, in rare form, she went to work. She introduced us to the staff and told them what she required of them. She then took me to my seat and when the tech came over to connect me to the machine, my wife called the doctor and said: "My husband is not a cripple. He's intelligent and everything that ya'll about to do to him needs to be explained first."

She then looked at me and said: "You will take notes and learn this machine and how to stick yourself within two weeks." I knew every button on the machine and, in 30 days, I learned how to stick myself since I was the only patient to do so. My diabetes was in check for the most part, but we knew I wouldn't last forever on dialysis so she started on her quest to get me a kidney. Within two and a half years, I received a duo transplant, a pancreas, and a kidney. From there, my life has changed.

Thanks to my wife, Nakita, and my children for fighting this battle with me and helping to save my life. I am forever grateful.

David Nelson was born in February 1969 in New Orleans, Louisiana. He is the oldest of nine children. Both of his parents are deceased.

David has been married to his lovely wife, Nakita, for over 20 years, and they have two children, which he adores. He was diagnosed with diabetes in his late 40s. His curiosity over where the disease came from led to him conducting further research on the disease.

David gathered the much-needed knowledge that allowed him to receive a duo transplant in 2.5 years of being on dialysis. Three and a half years later, David continues to do well with his duo transplant. He wanted to be a part of this book to share his journey and inform others that there is work to be done in the fight for a healthier you.

David considers his research "life knowledge that changed his life for the healthier good."

MY DIABETES JOURNEY
CARMEN WILLIAMS

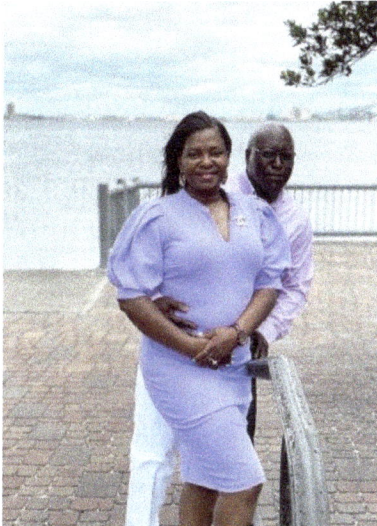

I was initially diagnosed in 2001. I was visiting with Dr. Broussard in Lake Charles, Louisiana, for a routine check-up. I had mentioned to her about my weight gain.

I weighed around 200 to 225 pounds. I was also extremely fatigued often. However, I honestly thought it was a part of the weight gain.

Having made the recent decision to get out of the Army, I assumed all of these were symptoms of depression. I figured the weight gain and fatigue were just a part of the adjustment process for me. After all, the career change from the Army to stay-at-home mom had my emotions on an all-time high.

When I expressed my concerns to Dr. Broussard, she ordered blood work. Shortly after the appointment, maybe a few days later, I was called in for a follow-up appointment and test results. This was the day my new reality was given to me and I was diagnosed as pre-diabetic!

I can recall this moment as if it was yesterday. I sat very still and in shock. My first thought was, "No way, not me!" I was under the impression that diabetics were people who just could not eat sweets and had issues with insulin. Those symptoms did not seem to fit me.

I gained weight and was tired, but I never expected this to be the cause. The doctor explained to me that going forward I would be taking a pill every day. I took the medicine as prescribed and followed all recommendations. I went into a crazy rage, determined to lose weight with the hopes that this would all just go away. However, it did not.

My A1C numbers stayed around 6.5-7.0 A1C. In three months, I went from pre-diabetic to diabetic. I was taking the medicine, working out and it was still not enough. My doctor increased my dosage from one pill a day to three! Receiving this news was extremely disappointing, to say the least.

Along with the increase came a heightened terror. Not knowing anyone with this diagnosis, I felt as if I was alone. I had no idea what to expect going forward. I kept working relentlessly on losing weight and stayed dedicated to my dieting. My doctor, along with my support system, helped me realize I could still live a good life. Diabetes was only a diagnosis and not a death sentence.

It is extremely vital to maintain your health. Stay up to date with your yearly wellness visits and do not be afraid to go more frequently if needed. This will allow you to catch the insulin resistance on time, which can increase the chances of reversal. Keep in mind, even if reversal is not possible, if you make the right lifestyle changes, things will get better.

Stay on your medications. Work out as much as possible. Re- evaluate your eating habits. If maintaining a healthy diet is a struggle, do not be afraid to ask your doctor for a nutritionist referral. As diabetes is more common than we think, many support groups are available if the journey becomes increasingly overwhelming.

Carmen Williams, 47, was born in Hope, Arkansas on December 28th, 1973. She has happily been married to Jerry Williams for six years. She is the daughter of Gloria Philpot and Raymond Johnson.

After serving in the United States Army from 1993-2000, she dedicated her time to her children. She now has five children ranging in ages 10 to 26.

She settled in Lake Charles, Louisiana, and recently relocated to Crosby, Texas. Her season in Lake Charles allowed her to obtain a degree in Industrial Instrumentation from Sowela Technical Community College. This degree led her to a successful 13-year career as a generator operator at Westlake Chemical. Although health issues led her to medical leave, she is still enjoying the fruits of her labor from mothering and working.

ENCOURAGEMENT

Having a positive mindset is always great for your overall health. I want to share some daily affirmations from my Facebook group page, **Conquering Diabetes**, which I invite you to join.

4 Daily Affirmations

DIABETES MADE BETTER, LLC

Repeat this to yourself daily:

1. Good riddance to decisions that do not support self-care, self-value, and self-worth.

2. I am the architect of my life. I build its foundation and choose its content.

3. My ability to conquer challenges is limitless.

4. Today, I abandon my old habits and take up new and more positive ones.

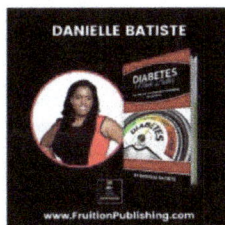

DANIELLE BATISTE

www.FruitionPublishing.com

We've Conquered This Disease

BY CHELSEA BATISTE

Having diabetes could be a struggle at first,
But we have to realize,
That if we eat healthier and fight harder,
It wouldn't control our lives.

You are not alone; there are many whom have it
And some cases worse than others,
No needle stick or patch on our arms could define
Our sisters and brothers.

A firm believer that if we do what's right
And supply our body's needs,
We all could stand up firm and shout:
"WE'VE CONQUERED THIS DISEASE."

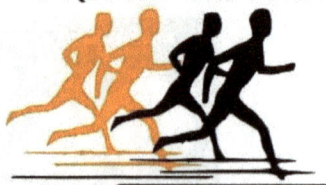

DIABETES AND COVID-19

I cannot end this book without addressing COVID-19 and diabetes.

Please be careful and mindful of your surroundings in this pandemic (at the time of this publication). Please wear your mask, take every precaution available, and stay safe. The COVID-19 vaccination is an important tool to protect the health and safety of citizens and end the pandemic which has taken a staggering toll on people living with diabetes.

My way of trying to help while educating myself is to not allow busyness, laziness, or fear to cause me to be complacent and not actively manage my diabetes. We all have choices and doing nothing is also a choice that carries consequences. I am not telling you to go get a vaccination, but I am telling you to be proactive and make educated decisions.

My personal choice was to be vaccinated and I received my two- dose COVID-19 vaccination with no side effects. Whatever you decide, please stay safe. ALWAYS wear your MASK, DISINFECT, and AVOID LARGE CROWDS. I chose to stay home because it is not only me I'm protecting, it's my whole family.

I told you that I would keep it real in this book and there is one thing I do not like to hear: that I can reverse diabetes by taking this or that.

I have beat diabetes because my A1C was below 7. Newsflash, I'm happy and ecstatic that you have done the work to get where you are with your A1C, but you still have the disease in your body and must remain vigilant. If you stop doing the right thing, you will find that the disease will return and perhaps worse than before.

How can you best help others with diabetes? By educating and empowering them to change their mindset and your best way to do that is by leading by example. No, it is not your job to tell them everything they are doing wrong or being the food police, but to lead by example and open the door to conversation. Diabetes is a serious chronic illness not to be taken lightly.

I constantly read and from my diabetes journey from diagnosis at age 39 to now age 47, there have been huge shifts and changes. Diabetes moves with you.

I'd rather share my experiences because the one thing that happens to me can help someone newly diagnosed and bring them clarity and peace of mind. We are in the fight together, so whatever I can share to lighten someone's burden, educate, and empower them is my mission and purpose.

A question I am often asked is "What is the problem?" The simple
answer is not enough people are taking the time to educate

themselves about this disease and think cutting a few things out will cure them.

I want to end by saying that I sincerely hope you love the information that we have shared and that I was able to do exactly what I set out to do: to educate and empower you on what diabetes is, what it can do, and what needs to be done to stay on top of it to not let it take control of our bodies like we have witnessed in so many people before us.

I enjoyed every bit of writing this book and I will be enjoying the next chapter of my life coaching diabetics on their mindset regarding this disease and continue to come out with great things for you to keep empowering yourself to conquer. We will not live for diabetes, but we will live despite this disease and we will live well. I love you guys and let us keep pushing.

<u>HYPOGLYCEMIA UNAWARENESS</u>

I wanted to add this chapter to my book after coming across this myself. I had read it many times before, but one thing is clear I personally never heard much talk about it and many are not even aware because they do not pay enough attention to their own bodies. Now to give you a little bit of meaning of what hypoglycemia unawareness is: you are constantly having low blood sugar episodes and this in turn can cause you to stop sensing the early warning signs, or you can be a diabetic as long as I have so you are missing the signs but please don't beat yourself up that's why this chapter is added to put everyone on notice about something simple we can all miss.

Now let's talk about our diet for hypoglycemia which I'm sure we all are doing great with but continue to put fresh vegetables, whole grains, and lots of protein. I'm just naming a few you get the picture.

One thing that would make a diabetic really into unawareness is if he or she consume alcohol. This in term will lower your ability to recognize any symptoms which will impair your liver's ability to release glucose when your blood sugar is too low. Now, you ask how long this might take will last as long as it takes your body to process that alcohol. Now I'm not saying alcohol increase hypoglycemia unawareness long erm unless its chronic and heavy drinking which can lead to permanent things like liver issues which is more sever hypoglycemia,

How to protect yourself:
1. More frequent blood glucose testing (fingerstick)
2. Work with your healthcare provider

www.Diatribe.org

Disclaimer: I'm here to educate but PLEASE CONSULT WITH YOUR DOCTOR ON EVERYTHING

-

MEET THE AUTHOR

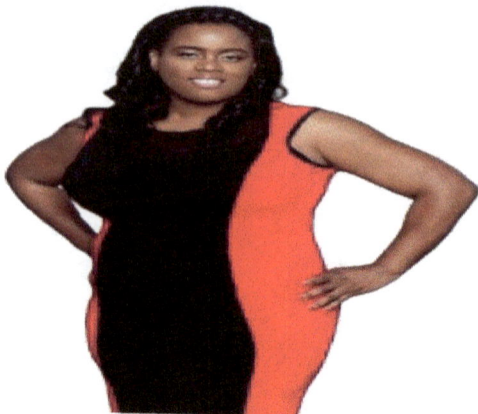

Best-Selling Author Danielle Batiste is a woman on a mission to improve the lives of diabetics everywhere and provide tools and resources for a better quality of life. The military veteran would like to eradicate the disease altogether. Why? Because after serving and protecting her country as a military service member, she found herself in a fight for her life. Danielle was diagnosed as a Type 2 Diabetic.

Effective management after diagnosis can be cumbersome, but Danielle reminds audiences that diabetes does not have to be a death sentence. In her book *Let Go My Glucose: Winning with Type 2*, Danielle chronicles her lifestyle journey after diabetes, the good and the bad:

When first diagnosed I went into denial because it was the easiest thing to do and the safest place to go, so I allowed my glucose levels to get out of control and I didn't have a clue on how to handle the dysfunction.

After going through this for a while I realized I can't live like this anymore. I was letting the disease win and that's not my nature.

I began learning everything on my own and the first thing I did was start learning my body, how it works, and how diabetes was affecting me.

I started paying more attention to what I ate, reading labels, and getting my correct numbers from my doctor.

What I hated most was pricking my finger and the way I had to live. The biggest thing for me was getting out there and exercising. I lost 40 pounds and that's when the fighting machine began. I knew then I wanted to help others.

Danielle has created an entire educational program for diabetes management and disease eradication which includes:

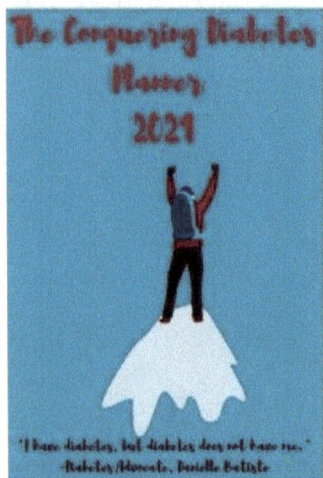

- The Conquering Diabetes Planner 2021

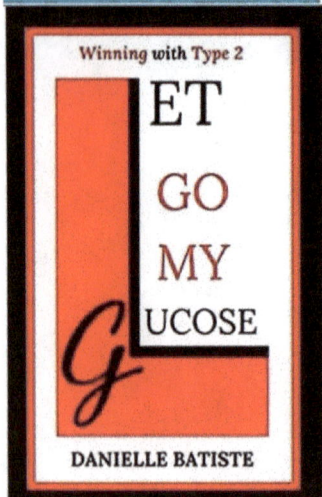

- LET GO MY GLUCOSE: Winning with Type 2

<u>SPECIAL THANKS</u>

A special thanks to the following people to be the first to support the publication of this book.

~ Danielle

- Jerome Bigham
- Mary Billingsley
- Jackie Gardner
- Pamela Garrison
- Melissa Glasper
- Sheldine Gordon
- Tracy Huffman
- Cintrell Hurst
- Hope Jackson
- Damien Jenkins-Bond
- Krystal Jones
- Marvelle Perrin
- Dorothy Powell
- Rosayliz MB
- Angie Siler
- Stacy Taylor

- Johnny Harris
- Nakita Harris
- Adriana Nelson
- Eduardo Nelson
- Charles Ricks
- Assata Nelson
- Raymond Johnson
- Candice Stokes
- Dominyck Harley
- Mekeri Williams

Please visit https://www.daniellebatiste.com/diabetes-made-better for more information and to connect with Danielle Batiste. On her website, she offers healthy recipes, tips and resources, and a quiz you can take to see if you are at risk. You do not have to fight this battle alone.